THE IMMUNE FITNESS PROJECT

FOOD ALLERGY RESILIENCE

DR DOUGLAS JONES, MD

DR NINA MARKOVIC KHAZE, PHD

IMMUNITY GROUP
AUSTRALIA

First published in Australia in 2023
by Immunity Group, Sydney, Australia

Paperback ISBN 978-0-6459793-0-5
E-book ISBN 978-0-6459793-1-2

For information, please contact: immunitygroupaustralia@proton.me

Printed and bound in Australia by
BA Printing & Publishing Services Pty. Ltd.
41 Sydenham Road, Brookvale NSW 2100
www.baprinting.com.au

A catalogue-in-publication entry is available from the National Library of Australia.

Disclaimer: The authors and publisher take no responsibility for any errors, omissions, or contradictions which may exist in the book. The information contained in this publication is for general information purposes only. It does not constitute or seek to provide any medical advice, including treatments for adverse food reactions or any other condition. Its primary purpose is to educate and raise awareness about allergies and microbiome health. If you require individually tailored advice, please consult your medical specialist or healthcare professional. The authors of this publication or the publisher are not liable for injuries or damage incurred by any person as a result of reading or following the information contained in this publication.

Book and cover design by Immunity Group Australia.

This book is dedicated to all the seekers of a healthy truth.

Contents

Your gut is a pillar
of your immunity.

Introductory remarks by Douglas Jones, MD, FAAAAI, FACAAI (USA)

When thinking of food allergies, many think of preventing an acute life-threatening event. The focus is on anaphylaxis. What does that really imply, though? It implies a chronic, every-minute-of-every-day experience as that is what it takes to prevent the acute reaction. It is a life and a lifestyle. It is one of restriction, often isolation, and can be taxing on the patient and the social community supporting the patient, provoking fear, and anxiety.

If we approach food allergy as solely a diagnosis, food avoidance, adrenaline usage, and hope, then I think we are really failing to see the bigger picture. It is so much more than that. Each person is an individual with uniqueness and past circumstances that led them to where they are today. We must take the whole person, including their community, into account when caring and serving those with food allergy and adverse reactions.

Emotional and spiritual aspects of dealing with food adverse reactions

The psychosocial, emotional, and spiritual impacts of adverse reactions to foods are often overlooked and underappreciated. It is a difficult thing to quantify, even if that is possible. Nevertheless, the ramifications are real. People with unpredictable chronic disorder are likely to experience depression and anxiety. The unknown diagnosis can be more debilitating to people than even a terminal diagnosis. Even though adverse reactions to foods can be diagnosed, the unknown or unpredictable nature of it weighs on people. The risk of being potentially life-threatening adds to the burden. I have seen personalities change as people are thrust into the food allergy life.

Interestingly, when I first started treating food allergies, my focus was like many - solely on the diagnosis, if adrenaline was needed and how many times, and getting the patient to safely eat the food.

While walking this journey with so many, I started noticing that as the patient and their community went through the food allergy treatment process, a surprise happened - personalities emerged, more eye contact and smiles were shared, and the weight on the shoulders became lighter. I gained a greater appreciation of the burden people were carrying once it was gone. Prior to that, I could not adequately discern the impact.

5 aspects of immune fitness

I do my best to meet the patient where they are on their journey. It is important to see where they have been and what has brought them to this point. Then, I want to know where they want to go. I see myself as a guide to help navigate the path to get them to that destination.

To do this, I must consider their overall fitness as a person. Fitness is not just physical. I have found that there are 5 key aspects of fitness:

1. **Social fitness** - what is the nature of their relationships? This could be family, friends, romantic relationships, colleagues, co-workers, strangers, and even pets. Are their relationships draining their energy or charging their battery?

2. **Mental fitness** - this encompasses their mindset, their self-awareness, and what they are putting into their mind - what are they consuming mentally?

3. **Emotional fitness** - what is the person's state of being? Are they carrying or storing emotional traumas? Are they stressed, anxious, or depressed? How do they respond to situations?

4. **Physical fitness** - what are they consuming to fuel their bodies? What is the quality and quantity that will comprise the building blocks of the cells of their body? Are they moving their bodies regularly in a way that is realistic for them? Are they allowing adequate rest and recovery?

5. **Spiritual fitness** - are they engaged with something bigger than them that is feeding their soul? Do they have a routine of prayer, meditation, or just silence with themselves?

This publication will provide some additional basic insights into some of those key innovative considerations that may not have been emphasised in times past. How do these concepts apply to those experiencing food adverse reactions and how can we develop resilience?

Be prepared, not scared.

Dr Douglas Jones MD

PART 1: Gut start your day

Gut health, as a pillar of human and immune fitness, is the new buzzword of the life sciences.

The word 'immunity', as it is being used today, was coined in the late Middle Ages from the Latin word *immunitas*, in reference to the protection from legal prosecution offered to Roman senators. Historically, immunity represents the body's ability to defend against or resist infections and diseases.

With the exponential growth of chronic health conditions, especially in societies with a modern diet, scientists worldwide have been researching the potential influence of gut health and microbiome on a person's overall health status. It has been found that gut health and microbiome can really impact immunity - in a myriad of ways, the fine details of which are still being studied.

Did you know?

Chronic and low-grade inflammation can turn into a silent killer and contribute to a range of disorders.

Allergies can develop at any age, including in adults.

1 in 10 Australian children and 1 in 20 adults have food allergies.

'Immunising' our supermarket shelves

In recent years, there has been a surge in the marketing of products claiming to support immunity and promote gut health. This includes a wide range of items, such as kombucha-style beverages, probiotic-rich yoghurts, vitamin-infused gummy candies, prebiotic-enriched breads, and a multitude of various supplements. For the average consumer, this plethora of choices can be bewildering.

Furthermore, this global trend of 'immunising' products on the supermarket shelves has coincided with the growth of scientific research papers into gut health, revealing new insights about our internal ecosystem.

Initial findings from different corners of the globe indicate that a highly diverse gut microbial environment, representing an individualised habitat for trillions of microbes residing in our intestines, may play a significant role in human health. There are also important microbial ecosystems on the skin and all mucosal linings – even in the lungs.

The exact mechanisms governing this diversification and how it should be managed remain less understood. For this reason, it is safe to say that a wide-ranging set of products that claim health benefits might be, at best, dubious. What does the widely used slogan 'support the immune system' even mean?

Comfort of an illusion

Yet, we continue to purchase and fill our pantries with such products. Does it make us feel better having them there? Is this our own comfort zone, knowing that we have ticked a box when it comes to our health without any deeper self-awareness and reflection, and before doing any real 'homework' on how to optimise our immunity from within?

One of the questions worth exploring is:

Can vitality and immunity optimisation be learned and developed through healthier habits?

We believe that it can. Immunity optimisation is a process and journey, full of unknowns. Nonetheless, clinical cases from the US indicate that modifying immunity and even potentially altering an individual's food allergy status can be achieved through a tailored, methodical, and scientific approach, adapted to each person's distinct health circumstances. Such an approach is known as oral immunotherapy. It involves administering escalating quantities of a food allergen while closely monitoring the patient's condition under medical supervision.

Oral immunotherapy

Oral immunotherapy (OIT), which has been practised in the US, Canada, in Europe, Singapore, the United Arab Emirates, and Israel over the past decade, has shown incredible results in practice for individuals living with food allergy. The European Academy of Allergy and Clinical Immunology calls OIT as being *currently the only available curative treatment for food allergy*. It is no longer a matter of contention that OIT works in changing the threshold a person may react to a food when allergic, but there are many studies that explore why and under what conditions OIT works *best*.

Having guided over 2,500 patients to food freedom over the last decade through a scientific-based approach–without requiring therapeutics in most instances–Dr Jones has devised a distinctive clinical method that melds OIT with microbiome diversification and specialised testing. His program, which has been embraced and customised to suit local conditions in various clinics worldwide, necessitates meticulous preparation of the gut for a transformative shift through a mindset change to start with.

Let's discuss now food allergy diagnostics and the risks associated with non-validated tests.

Non-validated allergy testing

Food allergy testing commonly involves skin prick tests. Tests measuring serum IgE levels that target specific foods, and their components are also common.

Emerging, but not yet widely available tests include basophil activation and epitope tests as the newest scientifically validated diagnostic tools for food adverse reactions, including allergies.

It is worth noting that some tests, despite their advertising, still lack validation. These tests do not consistently align with symptoms, while also lacking strong supporting evidence of their efficacy in diagnosing food allergies, intolerances, or sensitivities. Such tests include IgG tests, cytotoxic food testing, electrodermal tests, Vega and pulse testing, kinesiology, saliva and hair analysis, and flow cytometry assessing white blood cell morphology.

Non-validated allergy testing is not only confusing, but it can be expensive and lead to unforeseen outcomes that can derail one's immune fitness journey. There is a reason the tests are not validated.

Exponential growth of gut health concerns globally

Coping with gut health issues can present a daily challenge. Millions of individuals worldwide grapple with diverse gut health-related conditions, encompassing food sensitivities, inflammatory bowel syndrome (IBS), bloating, acid reflux, irregular bowel movements, and various chronic diseases. All these conditions necessitate specialised examination and interpretation. Scientists, clinicians, and researchers have identified a common thread among many of these ailments - an underlying inflammation triggered by various causes.

In the US, approximately 70 million people contend with digestive disorders, while in Australia, one in seven adults confronts distressing gut-related symptoms. While conventional approaches to managing these conditions primarily focus on putting out the fire, researchers are increasingly asking the following questions:

Is there something that individuals can adopt or incorporate into their daily routines to enhance their gut health and potentially even optimise their immunity?

Can we treat the root causes instead of managing the effects?

It's good to get messy.

Dr Alfred William Frankland (1912-2020), a British allergist and immunologist, who coined the hygiene hypothesis.

PART 2: Microbiome matters

The microbiome refers to the collection of microorganisms, including bacteria, viruses, fungi, and other microbes that live in and on the human body as well as in other environments, such as soil and water. However, when people commonly refer to the microbiome, they are often talking about *human microbiome*, which is the vast community of microorganisms that inhabit our bodies.

The human microbiome is most extensively studied in the gastrointestinal tract (the gut microbiome), but it also exists on the skin, in the mouth, and in various other organs and body systems. These microorganisms play a crucial role in maintaining human health and are involved in various physiological processes, including:

- **Digestion** - gut bacteria help to break down food and extract nutrients from it.
- **Immune system** - the microbiome interacts with the immune system and can influence its development and function.
- **Protection** - beneficial bacteria help protect against harmful pathogens by competing for resources and producing antimicrobial substances.
- **Synthesis of vitamins** - some gut bacteria can synthesise essential vitamins and nutrients.

- **Brain-gut connection** - emerging research suggests that the microbiome may influence brain function and behaviour, leading to the concept of the gut-brain axis.
- **Immune tolerance** - the microbiome is thought to play a role in immune tolerance, helping the body to distinguish between harmful invaders and harmless substances.

Changes in the composition and diversity of the microbiome have been associated with various health conditions, including obesity, autoimmune diseases, allergies, and gastrointestinal disorders. Researchers are continuing to explore the complex interactions between the microbiome and human health to better understand how the microbiome can be harnessed to promote wellbeing and treat or prevent diseases.

Pre-, pro- and postbiotics

- **Prebiotics** – they fuel probiotics. Top 5 prebiotic-rich foods are garlic, onions, leeks, Jerusalem artichokes and dandelion greens. High prebiotic fruits include bananas, watermelon, custard apples and grapefruit.

- **Probiotics** – fermented foods are rich in beneficial bacteria known as probiotics. These bacteria can improve digestion, boost immunity, and help maintain a healthy balance of gut microbiota.

- **Postbiotics** – substances generated as metabolic byproducts from beneficial probiotic bacteria during their growth and metabolic processes. These substances encompass a range of compounds, including short-chain fatty acids, peptides, enzymes, vitamins, organic acids, and other bioactive molecules.

The effects of alcohol on microbiome

Moderate and chronic alcohol consumption can have different impacts on the microbiome and overall health.

While moderate consumption might not have significantly detrimental effects for healthy individuals, chronic and heavy alcohol use is more likely to be harmful and lead to noticeable changes in the microbiome and related health issues.

Maternal microbiome

Researchers have found that maternal microbiota influences foetal development. Emerging studies examining the maternal-foetal interface tend to focus on maternal uterine-, gastrointestinal-, vaginal- and oral microbiota, as well as the endometrium and placental microbiota - both of which remain, at present, poorly understood.

It has become common knowledge that babies delivered via caesarean section (C-section) tend to develop food allergies and eczema more often than babies delivered vaginally. However, one Australian study led by the Murdoch Research Institute from Victoria did not find any significant difference between the two cohorts.

Babies born vaginally are certainly more exposed to maternal bacteria than those delivered via C-section. If, how and why that might influence the infant's predisposition towards developing food allergies later in life is still a scientific mystery and the subject of ongoing scientific enquiries.

The maternal microbiome certainly plays a role in the development of every infant's immune system.

Australia: the food allergy capital of the world

Australia has the highest prevalence of food allergies per capita in the world, with more than one million Australians being diagnosed with the condition. Furthermore, Australia has one of the highest C-section delivery rates among Organisation for Economic Co-operation and Development (OECD) countries - 38% of all women giving birth in Australia and 30% of women giving birth for the first time (2021 statistics), compared to the OECD average of 28%.

The United Kingdom comes second in terms of food allergic individuals per capita, with more than 1% of the total British population having been diagnosed (around 6 million people). In the US, around 20 million Americans reported having food allergies in 2021.

Food adverse reactions cost the Australian economy more than $7 billion per year, including in absences and lost productivity. In the UK and US, the cost is far higher.

There are many theories and assumptions as to why Australia is at the top of this list. Apart from the C-section hypothesis, other theories include Vitamin D deficiency among Australian pregnant women in particular; antibiotic overuse, including during pregnancy and shortly after birth; excessive cleanliness in our society; and the use of pesticides which make their way to the human food chain. There is no definitive answer as to why Australians have the highest rate of food adverse reactions per capita in the Western world.

Gut health is the newest line of enquiry in this field. Apart from environmental factors and genetics, it is increasingly believed that gut health plays a major role in inflammatory processes in the body. Even Australia's CSIRO, our national science agency, is working to deliver *a dietary strategy to promote a healthy and resilient gut microbiota during early life*. Its scientists are currently examining how the earliest stages of a baby's life, including the fermentation capability of infant gut microbiota during the weaning phase, might influence gut health resilience. The role of prebiotics (including Australian seaweed, for example), probiotics and postbiotics is also being assessed in many laboratory models in Australia and abroad, including studying their effect on gut microbiota.

For food allergies in particular, *Lactobacillus rhamnosus* (LGG) has been identified as a particularly beneficial probiotic that helps in reducing inflammation in the gut relating to food allergies. Microbial diversity in the gut is potentially the key to reducing chronic inflammation, offering benefits against many health conditions, including food allergies, but also dementia and many other conditions.

Vitamin D

Vitamin D may not be a vitamin at all. It is a hormone, or more accurately, a pro-hormone. It has many functions in the body. It was first noticed to play a role in bone health and that is where the original focus was centred. The reference ranges for what is considered normal in a person were based on the minimum amount of vitamin D needed to prevent rickets. Those ranges have not changed despite an explosion of scientific evidence showing the multiple roles of vitamin D, including vital functions in bone health, inflammation, immunity, skeletal muscle contraction, neuromuscular communication, and cardiovascular function. In terms of allergy and allergic or inflammatory conditions, vitamin D acts as an anti-inflammatory.

There are 2 main forms of vitamin D:

- **Vitamin D2 (ergocalciferol)** - found in some mushrooms and fortified foods
- **Vitamin D3 (cholecalciferol)** - found in certain animal-sourced foods like fatty fish, liver, and egg yolks. It is also the form of vitamin D that the skin synthesises when exposed to sunlight.

Ensuring sufficient levels of vitamin D is crucial for overall immune fitness. Sunlight serves as a natural source; however, factors such as sunscreen usage, indoor living, and geographical location can influence exposure to

UVB rays. Therefore, some individuals might need to rely on dietary sources and supplements. It is always advisable to seek professional guidance before incorporating any new supplements into your regimen.

Did you know?

Scientists studying Vitamin D deficiency and its various health effects found that people with low vitamin D levels often suffer from mood disorders, and allergies.

Vitamin D levels can be elevated by exposure to sunlight, consuming foods rich in vitamin D, or using supplements following advice from your healthcare professional.

Black seed oil (Nigella sativa)

Extracted from the seeds of the *Nigella sativa* plant, black seed oil has been historically valued in various cultures for its medicinal qualities. It has recently attracted attention for its potential ability to reduce inflammation, a property attributed to compounds such as thymoquinone present in the oil. Identified as the principal component in black seed oil, thymoquinone has demonstrated anti-inflammatory, antioxidant, and anti-cancer properties in numerous studies.

Preliminary research indicates that black seed oil potentially inhibits inflammatory substances like leukotrienes and prostaglandins, which play a pivotal role in inflammatory responses. For individuals dealing with chronic inflammatory diseases like rheumatoid arthritis, asthma, and inflammatory bowel disease, black seed oil presents a promising option, although conclusive benefits and dosage guidelines require further research.

Until more conclusive research is conducted, including scientifically validated human clinical trials, individuals should proceed with caution and seek professional healthcare advice regarding its use and safety, as well as any potential drug interactions. Selecting premium products from trustworthy suppliers is also essential.

Fibre

What is fibre? The word comes from the Medieval Latin *fibra*, meaning 'filament, entrails' and the Latin word *filum*, meaning 'a string, or thread'.

Fibre is a type of carbohydrate that is indigestible in the small intestine. Plant foods contain fibre which cannot be completely broken down by human digestive enzymes. Fibre provides fuel for beneficial bacteria, potentially making the human gut more resilient. Certain types of fibre can serve as prebiotics, hence their designation as 'food' for good gut microbes.

There are 2 types of fibre, soluble and insoluble.

Soluble fibre forms a gel-like substance in water. In this form, it can help reduce glucose and cholesterol levels. It can help to manage diarrhoea by absorbing water and forming a gel. Foods that contain soluble fibre include barley, oats, apples, carrots, citrus fruits, beans, peas and psyllium.

Insoluble fibre does not dissolve in water and passes undigested through the gastrointestinal tract. It can help prevent constipation as it adds bulk to human stool and promotes the movement of material through the digestive system. Foods that contain insoluble fibre include nuts, seeds, wheat bran, whole-wheat flour, beans, and vegetables such as celery, cabbage, green beans, potatoes, and cauliflower.

Benefits

The benefits of dietary fibre are numerous and still studied. Consuming a fibre-rich diet can help prevent inflammation and chronic conditions such as type 2 diabetes and might also assist in weight regulation.

Did you know?

Fibre exclusively exists in plant-based sources and is entirely absent in meat and animal products.

Most people don't consume the minimum recommended quantity of fibre.

Insufficient fibre consumption can lead to a range of health problems, including digestive issues and constipation.

Omega-3 fatty acids

Omega-3 fatty acids are a variety of polyunsaturated fats that the human body requires for its optimal immune fitness. Our bodies cannot produce Omega-3 fatty acids on their own, so we need to consume Omega-3 rich dietary sources. There are 3 main types of these fatty acids:

- **Alpha-linolenic acid (ALA):** primarily sourced from plants, such as basil seeds, flaxseeds, chia seeds, walnuts, and canola oil. It's classified as an essential fatty acid because the human body cannot synthesise it and must obtain it from food.

- **Eicosapentaenoic acid (EPA):** EPA is predominantly found in marine organisms, especially in fatty fish like salmon, mackerel, and sardines. It is renowned for its anti-inflammatory attributes and is commonly linked to cardiovascular health.

- **Docosahexaenoic acid (DHA):** DHA is abundant in marine life, particularly in fatty fish. It plays a pivotal role in brain development and function, particularly during pregnancy and infancy. Additionally, DHA is essential for maintaining optimal vision and a healthy nervous system.

Resistant starch

Regular (simple) starch, also known as amylum, belongs to the family of complex carbohydrates and consists of glucose molecules. The main starches are barley starch, cassava starch, corn starch, maize starch, pea starch, potato starch, rice starch, sorghum starch, tapioca starch, and wheat starch. The US is the world's largest producer of maize starch, while the European Union produces mostly potato and wheat starch.

Apart from offering nutritional benefits, starch has a wide range of industrial applications. It is used in the food industry to enhance product shelf life, in the chemical industry, and in the production of industrial adhesives, cosmetic products, paper, and oral pharmaceuticals. Common foods containing starch include potatoes, sweet potatoes, cereal grains (such as wheat, corn, barley, and rice), legumes (like peas, chickpeas, and beans), immature fruits and vegetables, turmeric, and ginger. Fruits and vegetables store energy in the form of starch.

Starchy foods provide humans with energy and serve as a nutritious dietary source. While most starches are broken down in the human small intestine into sugar, causing an insulin spike, resistant starch plays a crucial role in promoting a healthy gut microbiome. Resistant starch is a type of dietary fibre, specifically a homo-polysaccharide that is water-insoluble. It resists digestion and undergoes fermentation by intestinal bacteria in the large intestine. This fermentation process releases short-chain fatty acids, such as butyrate, acetate, and propionate, which can have numerous health benefits. Butyrate feeds the cells lining the colon and can help prevent increased intestinal permeability.

Resistant starch serves as a substrate for fermentation by gut bacteria in the colon, while also enhancing the integrity of the gut barrier. It is naturally found in:

- green bananas and raw potatoes
- certain whole grains (oats and barley)
- the fibrous cell walls of plants
- cooked and cooled starchy vegetables, such as squash, beans, and legumes.

The quantity of resistant starch found in these foods can fluctuate based on variables such as cooking techniques and the stage of ripening.

Did you know?

Resistant starch aids in reducing the abundance of potentially pathogenic bacteria, which may especially be important in pregnancy. It may also help reduce the risk of inflammation and various gastrointestinal disorders, improve insulin sensitivity and digestion, and lower blood fats.

Consuming foods rich in resistant starch daily can help diversify the microbiota and promote the growth of beneficial bacteria in the gut.

Fermented foods

Fermentation is a metabolic process that converts simple carbohydrates into organic acids or alcohol using microorganisms (yeast or bacteria) with little or no oxygen. In many cultures, fermentation has traditionally been used to make alcoholic beverages and to extend the shelf life of foods, especially in winter months.

The fermentation process may create good bacteria that act as probiotics in the gut. Fermentation makes lactose easier to digest. The acids or alcohols produced act as natural preservatives and contribute to the unique flavours of fermented foods. Including fermented foods in the diet can be beneficial for maintaining a healthy gut microbiota and improving overall health.

Benefits for human health and microbiota

- **Nutrient absorption** – fermentation breaks down compounds called antinutrients, which can interfere with the absorption of nutrients. Eating fermented foods can improve nutrient absorption.
- **Vitamin synthesis** – some fermented foods are excellent sources of vitamins, especially B-

vitamins, as fermentation can increase the levels of these vitamins.

- **Bioavailability of compounds** – fermentation can increase the bioavailability of bioactive compounds and antioxidants, which are beneficial to human health.
- **Digestive health** – consuming fermented foods can help maintain a balanced gut flora, which is essential for digestive health. It may alleviate symptoms of irritable bowel syndrome, constipation, and diarrhoea.
- **Immune system boost** – a healthy gut microbiota contributes to optimal immune system function. Regular consumption of fermented foods can contribute to overall immunity.
- **Mental health** – there is a growing body of evidence suggesting a connection between gut health and mental health, known as the gut-brain axis. Consuming fermented foods might positively affect mental wellbeing.

Examples of fermented foods

- Yoghurt – fermented milk product, rich in probiotics.
- Sauerkraut – fermented cabbage, high in fibre and vitamins.
- Kimchi – Korean fermented vegetables, rich in vitamins A and C.

- Kombucha – fermented tea, rich in beneficial probiotics.
- Tempeh – fermented soybean product, which is a good source of protein and various nutrients.

Food allergy families are similar; the difference lies in individual responses to the newly diagnosed condition.

PART 3: Food allergy journey

For those unfamiliar with the terms 'food allergy', 'anaphylaxis' and 'food adverse reactions' - as are many food allergy parents before discovering their child's potentially life-threatening food adverse condition, or individuals who have developed a food allergy later in life - a brief overview of the considerations that guide a food allergy life might improve understanding of this growing public health issue.

Food allergy families face similar challenges, difficulties and fears that are quite common on their food allergy journey. Every food allergic individual's health status differs, as do their comorbidities. Yet, the diagnosis of a food allergy places a heavy burden on all food allergy patients and their carers. It adversely affects each family's quality of life, as reported in many surveys, and confirmed by clinical studies internationally.

Discovering food allergy: ground zero

Food allergy journeys are highly individualised and personal for each family, patient, and their immediate community. The one common characteristic is the shock of discovering the food allergy, followed by an enquiry stage and an eventual acceptance of the condition, whether temporary or permanent.

It is not uncommon for food allergy parents or individuals to develop mental health conditions, including but not limited to anxiety, depression, and paranoia, or for pre-existing conditions to deteriorate. Research has also shown that most food allergy families generally report their self-limiting life experiences and living in daily fear from accidental potentially life-threatening exposures.

Examples familiar to all food allergy families include self-exclusion from social and community events, family gatherings and even public spaces such as playgrounds or playcentres, and avoiding air travel or temporary accommodation, even for a holiday. The burden of living with food allergies is mitigated by families through a degree of self-isolation, avoiding cross-contamination and making sure that safe food spaces are always available.

The following section describes the various stages in the food allergy journey, starting with discovering food allergies in infants. Each stage of development presents a specific set of challenges for food allergy children and their caregivers.

Discovering food allergies in infants

Despite the early cues that some babies experience, including a variety of gastrointestinal symptoms; blood-stained and explosive, mucous stools; and severe skin rashes or eczema, primary caregivers usually discover their child's food allergy through a moderate to severe adverse reaction.

Having a baby diagnosed with a food adverse condition can be frightening. Introducing new foods or even trying baby milk formula for the first time can quickly become a parent's worst nightmare if it is accompanied by a food adverse reaction. Primary caregivers, in particular mothers, experience under-reported or unrecognised anxiety related symptoms associated with the fear of feeding their baby anything new.

A failure to thrive occurs in many allergic babies. Breastfeeding mothers usually modify their diet to prevent the allergen passing through their milk to the baby and work hard to maintain their milk supply as long as possible. For formula-fed babies, options are more limited, especially if babies refuse to accept amino acid or hydrolysed protein formulas.

The concept of safe spaces

It is not uncommon for primary carers of food allergic infants to trial new foods inside their GP's office, in a carpark near their local hospital's emergency department or in other spaces where they feel safer to manage any food adverse reaction. It is common for food allergy families, who might be experiencing fear and anxiety in silence, to seek out 'safe spaces', such as an uncontaminated living space, or a play zone or activity where their child is least likely to encounter a potentially life-threatening allergen. A home free from their child's allergen becomes the safest space for food allergy families.

Safe touch

In babies who have eczema, atopic dermatitis and food allergies, safe touch becomes problematic, especially in larger families. It is not uncommon for mothers to avoid touching or kissing their food allergic babies to prevent any skin flare-up. There are some estimates that around a third of infants with food allergies have eczema-prone skin. Changes in weather, such as humidity, may impact a baby's skin microbiome.

It is important to keep the allergic infant's skin as intact as possible, and to keep infants well-hydrated during the day and dressed in low-irritant and hypoallergenic clothes made from natural bamboo or pure cotton material. Textile cotton dermatitis occurs when a person reacts to the material used to produce the clothing but is more frequently a contact allergy to chemical additives used to process the fabric.

The early introduction of allergens

Although research has shown that introducing allergens early in infancy might help prevent food allergies later in life, infants with diagnosed food allergies are less likely to try a variety of new foods and textures due to parental fears that the child will experience a food adverse reaction. Their socialisation with other infants, being in public places, or their participation in early infancy activities are likely to be more limited than is the case for children living without food allergies.

Toddlers with food allergies

Primary caregivers of toddlers with food allergies must always remain vigilant. Toddlers are always keen to explore, but with food allergic children, any accidental ingestion of foods that may contain a potentially life-threatening allergen adds to the complexities of parenthood. Safe spaces and safe touch are often compromised in the toddler development stage. Toddlers with food allergies who attend day care are more likely to experience accidental exposures requiring emergency management of anaphylaxis, than those in more confined care arrangements.

School-age children and food allergies

Starting school for children with food allergies leads to conversations with the school management, teachers and health professionals involved in student care. School-age children who experience food adverse reactions are often bullied, with at least 40% of food allergic students reporting bullying at school because of their condition. Social exclusion is also an aspect of the food allergy journey for many school-age children and their families, whether initiated by peers or self-isolation, as it becomes difficult to manage social events involving food.

School camps with food allergies

Although all activities present challenges for food allergy families and individuals, school camps can cause an additional level of stress and anxiety. Still, it is important for all students to be included in school activities, including camps. Maintaining the delicate balance between safety and the emotional, physical, and social developmental aspects of food allergic children becomes an art for all individuals on the food allergy journey.

Puberty and food allergies

In puberty, the food allergy journey becomes more problematic with hormonal changes. Socially, teenagers tend to experiment more and take unnecessary risks, including with food. Of all the age groups, apart from toddlers, teenagers can have the highest incidence of food adverse reactions.

Eating out with food allergies

All food allergy families pause when it comes to eating out. Primary caregivers usually need to make pre-arranged meals or organise special meals in advance with the venue for their family members with food allergies. Still, exposures happen frequently when eating out, including fatalities. It is difficult to balance food and eating out being such a significant part of life.

Labelling laws also differ greatly between countries, which makes eating out for families and individuals with food allergies quite problematic - especially while travelling.

Babysitting and food allergies

For many families with food allergies, babysitting is an uncomfortable concept. Primary caregivers are almost always the most in tune with the needs of their food-allergic children. A babysitter can be a family member, friend, or a stranger. The main consideration regarding babysitting and food allergies is whether the person undertaking this important task is knowledgeable about using epinephrine auto-injectors, whether they will recognise any allergic reaction quickly enough, and how fast they will respond to any emergency.

Food freedom journey and parenting

Approaches developed by Dr Jones in clinical practice in the US that aim to retrain immunity not to recognise an allergen as enemy require strict observation. These methods involve diligent adherence to a structured routine, which must be maintained daily. Central to the success of these approaches is the diversification of the microbiome, a crucial element of the program.

While preparing the gut for improved health can be a time-consuming process, the benefits far outweigh any inconveniences. Parenting children undergoing OIT with microbiome diversification can be highly rewarding, as parents dedicate themselves to helping their child flourish. This journey is deeply personal, heavily influenced by the 5 facets of immune fitness.

Food allergy community

Over the past two decades, parents from all over the world have started to create informal and formal networks including online communities, not-for-profit organisations and virtual as well as physical social support groups for knowledge sharing, education, socialisation, and validation of their highly subjective experiences.

Advocacy networks in the food allergy realm are rapidly expanding, including in Australia. Global campaigns are resulting in architectural icons all over the world being lit up in teal - the colour representing food allergy awareness. Sydney Town Hall became the inaugural building outside North America to join the Turn it Teal initiative, which was started by American mother, Stephanie Lowe.

Some parents and carers change their entire careers and adopt new business ventures, such as selling allergy-friendly products, creating health food shop items (for example, yeast-free breads), or even investing in high-quality research, diagnostics, and medical treatments for improving food allergies. Together, and separately from the medical and scientific community, these individuals seek to break new ground and get to the bottom of the medical and social problem of food allergies.

Others go a step further and lobby policy-makers for legislative changes, better access to services and life-saving devices such as adrenaline autoinjectors, and more accurate diagnostic tools to diagnose and treat food allergies.

One's food allergy journey can be a path towards food freedom which is possible within a proven scientific framework and personalised approach.

PART 4: Meet your food allergen

Food allergies should not be confused with sensitivities or intolerances to food. In this section, we will discuss cow's milk allergy, egg allergy, peanut allergy, tree nut allergy, seed allergy, seafood allergy, and alpha-gal allergy. Please note that this is not a comprehensive list of allergens. Food allergy symptoms can manifest at any age.

Cow's milk allergy

An allergy to cow's milk protein (CMPA) occurs when the immune system reacts to one or several proteins present in cow's milk. This allergy is among the most prevalent of food allergies in children, with symptoms varying from mild reactions, such as hives and slight abdominal discomfort, to severe ones like anaphylaxis. Reactions can be classified into 2 types: IgE mediated and non-IgE mediated (e.g. FPIES). IgE mediated allergies are generally immediate and more intense and may result in multi-organ system anaphylaxis, while the latter are usually delayed, presenting as chronic conditions like eczema or gastrointestinal problems.

While there is no definitive data on the exact prevalence of CMPA in Australia, it is estimated to affect approximately 2 to 3% of infants. Notably, a significant number of children tend to outgrow this allergy by the time they are 3 to 5 years old, and 80% by the age of 16. The reported prevalence can vary, depending on the definitions applied, the demographics studied, and the method of data collection.

Managing an IgE-mediated dairy allergy can be complex due to the widespread inclusion of milk in numerous products, such as cosmetics, soaps, creams, and nutritional items.

Did you know?

A common misconception is that people allergic to dairy can safely consume lactose-free ingredients. Lactose is a sugar present in milk, while dairy can comprise more than 20 different proteins. Lactose intolerance often arises from an individual's insufficient enzymes in the small intestine to digest milk sugar, which makes up anywhere from 2 to 8% of milk content.

Egg allergy

Egg allergy is a common food allergy, especially among children. This allergy arises when the immune system abnormally responds to the proteins found in eggs, perceiving them as threats. Subsequently, the immune system releases chemicals like histamine to fight these proteins, resulting in allergic symptoms.

While egg allergies are more frequent in children, a significant number tend to outgrow the allergy as they age. Determining the precise prevalence of egg allergies in Australia is challenging, but various studies and surveys indicate that around 9% of infants and young children are affected. The reported prevalence can fluctuate depending on the data source, and not every individual sensitised to egg proteins will display clinical symptoms.

Did you know?

A common myth relating to egg allergy is that individuals who are allergic to egg white proteins can still consume egg yolk. Have you ever tried to completely separate the egg white from the egg yolk? Another myth is that egg allergic individuals are also allergic to chicken meat.

Peanut allergy

In the US, peanut is among the top 3 food allergens, apart from milk and egg allergy. It comes as no surprise that a lot of resources being invested in clinical trials relating to treating and potentially reversing peanut allergy, from companies aiming to develop vaccines, to those making desensitisation patchs, lollies, pills and even a toothpaste.

A peanut allergy arises when the immune system mistakenly recognises peanuts as harmful, leading to an allergic reaction. Compared to some other food allergies, like those to milk or eggs, peanut allergy is often more persistent, with fewer individuals outgrowing them.

In Australia, there is a growing concern regarding peanut allergy, as its prevalence has been on the rise. Research suggests that around 3% of children in Australia are affected, making it one of the most prevalent food allergies in the nation. Nonetheless, it is important to acknowledge that reported rates can differ depending on the criteria for diagnosis, the demographic studied, and the method of data collection. Those with a peanut allergy need to exercise caution, meticulously read food labels, and be aware of the potential risk of cross-contamination.

Peanuts are regularly found in many cosmetic products, confectionary and in sauces, oils, and household hygiene products.

Some individuals with peanut allergies exhibit a high sensitivity to airborne peanut particles. Air travel is particularly risky for those individuals.

Did you know?

An IgE-mediated peanut allergy is different from tree nut allergies. Peanuts belong to the legume family and grow underground, possessing proteins that are significantly different from those present in tree nuts.

Tree nut allergy

All nuts are not created equal! Each nut is unique.

Tree nut allergy is a widespread food allergy, characterised by the immune system abnormally responding to proteins in tree nuts. These nuts include almonds, cashews, walnuts, hazelnuts, pine nuts and pistachios, among others. When exposed, the immune system perceives these proteins as threats, and initiates an allergic reaction.

Compared to milk or egg allergies, tree nut allergy tends to be more enduring, with many individuals experiencing it throughout their lives, though some might outgrow it. Cross-reactivity can also occur, where individuals allergic to one type of tree nut may react to others they haven't been exposed to before. There are many non-food sources of tree nuts, including cosmetics, alcoholic beverages, beanbags, sandblasting materials, and sunscreens.

In Canada, tree nuts are listed as priority allergens (the foods that cause most allergic reactions). They include almonds, Brazil nuts, cashews, hazelnuts, macadamia nuts, pecans, pine nuts, pistachios, and walnuts.

In Australia, an allergy to tree nuts is a notable health concern. Research indicates that it affects approximately

2% of children, making it one of the more common food allergies among the young population in the country.

Did you know?

People allergic to tree nuts may not be allergic to coconut. A coconut is not a nut but a seed of a fruit.

Seeds allergy

Allergies to seeds, while less frequent compared to other food allergies, can trigger severe and potentially fatal reactions in susceptible individuals. Common culprits include seeds such as sesame, sunflower, poppy, mustard, and chia. Many baking products contain sesame seeds. Sesame is an allergen that contains protein and lipid allergens, which is a unique feature not found in other allergenic foods.

Seed allergies occur when the immune system mistakenly recognises seed proteins as harmful, prompting an immune response and resulting in allergic symptoms. In the context of Australia, allergies to sesame seeds are relatively more prevalent compared to other seeds. However, there is a lack of comprehensive documentation on the prevalence of seed allergies, making them less well-characterised than allergies to peanuts, tree nuts, eggs, or milk.

Current data indicates that the prevalence of sesame seed allergy in the Australian population is estimated to range between 0.1% and 0.2%, although this figure may vary, and the prevalence of allergies to other seeds remains somewhat ambiguous.

Did you know?

People with an allergy to one seed type are not necessarily allergic to other seeds.

Seafood allergy

Seafood allergy is characterised by an exaggerated immune response to proteins present in both shellfish and finned fish. Individuals with this allergy respond to proteins located in the muscle tissues of these marine creatures, and for some, merely inhaling vapours from cooking seafood may trigger a reaction.

Seafood can be primarily classified into 2 categories: shellfish, which includes crustaceans (for example, shrimp, crab, lobster) and molluscs (for example, clams, mussels, oysters, scallops), and finned fish, comprising species like tuna, salmon, and snapper. Individuals could be allergic to either or both categories.

In the context of Australia, allergies to seafood are notably prevalent. Studies reveal that around 2.5% of the Australian population claim to have a seafood allergy diagnosed by a medical professional, making it one of the predominant causes of food allergies for both adults and children in the country.

Did you know?

A prevalent myth about shellfish allergies is the belief that an allergy to shellfish or seafood implies an allergy to iodine as well. There is no association with shellfish allergy and iodine.

Alpha-gal allergy

Alpha-gal allergy, alternatively termed mammalian meat allergy, is an allergic reaction to galactose-alpha-1,3-galactose (alpha-gal), a sugar molecule found in the meat of most mammals, excluding primates (humans included). The primary cause of sensitisation to alpha-gal is bites from specific tick species, with the lone star tick (*Amblyomma americanum*), mainly found in the southeastern US, being the most notable. Nonetheless, various tick species globally, including those present in Australia, can induce this allergy.

Individuals with an alpha-gal allergy may exhibit a range of symptoms, encompassing hives, itching, abdominal discomfort, and in severe instances, anaphylaxis – a potentially fatal allergic reaction. A distinctive characteristic of this allergy is the delayed onset of symptoms, which often emerge several hours after ingesting mammalian meat such as beef, pork, or lamb. This delayed response sets it apart from most food allergies, where symptoms typically appear shortly after consumption.

There have been documented cases of alpha-gal allergy in Australia, predominantly in areas with a high concentration of ticks. However, establishing a precise prevalence rate of alpha-gal allergy in the country proves challenging due to the lack of comprehensive documentation. Recorded cases are notably present in regions with increased tick activity, including the coastal areas of NSW and Queensland.

In 2007, Australian physician, Clinical Professor Sheryl van Nunen became the first immunologist in the world to describe in a published paper the association between the mammalian meat allergy and ticks.

In her work, van Nunen found that Australia has the highest prevalence of mammalian meat allergy and tick anaphylaxis in the world. In 2021, Professor van Nunen was awarded the Order of Australia Medal (OAM) for service to medicine, particularly to allergy and clinical immunology.

Did you know?

Contrary to what is commonly and mistakenly assumed, the red meat allergy diverges from other food allergies in that it is triggered by a carbohydrate, not a protein.

It is also not a plot by vegans or vegetarians to destroy our meat industry!

It's good to focus on one step at the time.

PART 5: Live your best life now

The Immune Fitness and food allergy resilience concepts which were explored in this publication aim to inspire everyone to immediately work on pursuing their optimal life through education, self-discipline, and a dedicated commitment to daily improvement.

Formulating one's approach to strengthening gut health and diversifying the microbiome could include:

• developing a personal and individualised strategy for crafting one's own immune fitness and food allergy resilience map

• harbouring a mindset focused on health success and disseminating uplifting success stories to others

• undergoing scientifically validated testing for adverse food reactions

• prioritising holistic and nutritious eating, devoid of pesticides, artificial colours, and additives

• maintaining mindfulness regarding the importance of preserving healthy gut microflora within the body

• being conscious about the need to adopt healthy sleep patterns and managing stress levels, and

• ensuring the skin remains intact and eczema is controlled.

The emotional and spiritual facets of an individual's immune fitness should be considered when crafting one's gut health initiative.

Observing a daily, intelligent, and uncompromising approach towards one's health objectives is necessary.

Everybody's immune fitness and food allergy resilience goals can be perfected through regular practice and adaptation.

By working from the inside out and embarking on a path of learning and change, transformation can be achieved towards a healthier, happier, and the utmost version of oneself, which every individual deserves.

ACKNOWLEDGEMENTS

We would like to acknowledge and pay our respects to the Traditional Custodians of the land of the First Nations peoples from which we are writing: the Indian Nations of Utah, USA, and the Gayamagal People of the Eora Nation in Australia - including their Elders and leaders, past, present and emerging.

We extend our gratitude to all individuals who have contributed to this publication.

Ideas presented here are designed to serve as a widely engaging discussion tool that identifies strategies for optimising gut health. This discussion is titled *The Immune fitness project. Food allergy resilience* because the quest to enhance one's health and diversify microbiome is highly personal and individualised.

This publication does not intend to offer medical or health advice to treat any condition, either diagnosed or perceived. Instead, it seeks to serve as a conversation starter for anyone interested in topics related to immunity, allergies, and gut health in a broader context.

The authors of this book, Dr Douglas Jones, an American Board-certified allergist/immunologist from the United States (US), and Dr Nina Markovic Khaze, a specialised researcher from Australia, hope that the content within these pages will be of assistance in charting one's course towards a personalised immune fitness and food allergy resilience.

We hope that this publication will make a modest contribution to raising general awareness about the importance of gut health in optimising immunity, including the microbiome's role in preventing and potentially reversing adverse food conditions. Every person owns their individual gut health project. Let these reflections serve as a guide toward fortifying one's immune defences and guarding against any future complacency. May the journey of transformation begin here with us today.

IMMUNITY GROUP
AUSTRALIA

You can follow Dr Jones on Instagram @drdouglasjones

You can follow Immunity Group Australia on
YouTube @ImmunityGroup
Instagram @immunity.group.australia

Printed in Australia by
BA Printing & Publishing Services Pty. Ltd.
41 Sydenham Road, Brookvale NSW 2100
sales@baprinting.com.au

www.ingramcontent.com/pod-product-compliance
Lightning Source LLC
LaVergne TN
LVHW022026200926
848481LV00007B/2563
* 9 7 8 0 6 4 5 9 7 9 3 0 5 *